Headache is a Biological Conflict

Andrea Taddei

Headache is a Biological Conflict
Copyright © 2012 Andrea Taddei. All rights reserved.

ISBN-13: 978-1481143707
ISBN-10: 1481143700

Cover photo: www.istockphoto.com

To Matilde

CONTENTS

Andrea Taddei

FOREWORD

The Germanic New Medicine® discovered by Dr. Ryke Geerd Hamer and systematized in the 5 Biological Laws represents a change in the understanding of what is commonly called a disease.

Through his studies, Dr. R.G. Hamer, came to the conclusion that the disease processes are not "errors of nature" but rather Significant Biological Programs of Nature stemming from sudden and dramatic events.

This book was written with the intent of shedding light on the understanding of the 5 Biological Laws, for those looking for and wanting to understand the issue fully; the study of matter and the spirit, whether reflective, critical and scientific, is up to the reader.

For a correct diffusion of the authentic Germanic New Medicine® and studies related to the discoveries of Dr. Hamer, please refer to the reading of the Testament for a New Medical and Scientific Table of Dr. Ryke Geerd Hamer.

Andrea Taddei

All truth passes through three stages.

First, it is ridiculed.

Second, it is violently opposed.

Third, it is accepted as being self-evident.

Arthur Schopenhauer

Andrea Taddei

1. AN OLD VISION

At a certain stage of my life, I live a dramatic experience, that suddenly, catches me off-guard, I never thought such a thing could happen to me, in that moment, I am speechless, I am bewildered.

I'm freezing, my hands are very cold, and in the following minutes, hours, days, I can't help thinking about that thing that happened to me, so intensely, so unexpectedly, I cannot think of anything else, I say to myself, I want to sort this thing out! But now I can't, I keep thinking about how to get out of this, I can't sleep these days, I always wake up around 2 or 3 am.

I found the solution! I will do such and such, settle everything now! I'm going to fix it.

I've just got back, I am happy, I feel relieved at last! But now I'm a little tired, I'm very nearly going to bed without eating, what a hard time have I been through! Today has been a busy day!

The day after

I did not hear the alarm, it is eleven o'clock am but I'm really tired, I feel I'm running a temperature, my body aches, especially my legs, I cannot even get up,as if a truck had run me over.

It is 4:30 pm, I am in my doctor's waiting room, the door opens and I get in.

P.: Good afternoon Doctor!

D.: Good afternoon. How can I help you?

P.: I believe I caught 'flu.

D.: Please come closer so I can visit you, this is the time, it's virus season, November has come.

P.: How unlucky! You know Doctor, now that everything is going right, I feel so sick!

D.: Do not worry, this is just a seasonal disease, the whole city is in bed. Take this and get some rest for the next three days.

P.: Thank you Doctor!

2. THE 5 BIOLOGICAL LAWS

1st Biological Law of Nature

1st Criterion: every Significant Biological Special Programs of Nature (SBS) originates from DHS (Dirk Hamer Syndrome), with an unexpected conflict shock, acute and dramatic, lived intensely and with a feeling of isolation. Starting from DHS, every SBS manifests itself simultaneously on three levels: psyche, brain, organ.

2nd Criterion: DHS determines the location of the SBS both at brain level, the so-called Hamer Focus, and at organ level where it causes an organic alteration.

3rd Criterion: the course of the SBS runs synchronously on all three levels (psyche, brain and organ), from DHS to the resolution of the conflict (CL), including epi-crisis (CE) at the top of the Post-Conflict phase (PCL) until normal level is restored (normotonia).

As shown in the picture, we have a line that represents time passing by: it can be shown in seconds, minutes, hours, days, months or years, according to the shock occurred.

$$\xrightarrow{\hspace{8cm}} \text{time}$$

Above this line the sympathetic nervous system - also called orthosympathetic - is shown. (see Appendix)

Sympathicotonia

$$\xrightarrow{\hspace{8cm}} t$$

Under the timeline the parasympathetic nervous system is shown.

$$\xrightarrow{\hspace{8cm}} t$$

Vagotonia

Usually we are in a status of normotonia.

$$\xrightarrow{\hspace{8cm}} t$$

that is to say we physiologically fluctuate from a sympathetic nervous system activation to the parasympathetic nervous system activation: it is the day-night rhythm and the rest-activity rhythm.

During this normotonia - this is quite normal- an acute, unexpected, sudden, dramatic event may occur, which catches me off-guard and I live it as a state of isolation.

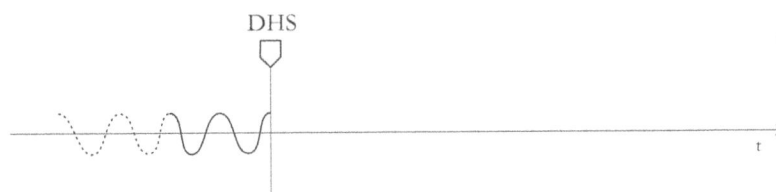

This event (DHS) represents the beginning of a cascade of immediate modifications that will occur simultaneously and instantly at three levels: at a psychic level I will have the memory of the biological conflict (DHS), at brain level, there will be an activation of the cerebral areas (HH-Hamer Focus) that are connected to the event experienced, while at an organ or bowel level, there will be some functional and structural modifications still connected to the event.

The DHS is a biological and not a psychological event.

The living organism should react in an optimal way and straight away to this event, as there is a risk for its safety, its own existence or the existence of the group to which it belongs.

2rd Biological Law of Nature

All Special Programs with the Biological Sense(SBS) consist of two phases, provided that you get to the solution of the conflict.

The 2nd Biological Law describes the Significant Biological Special Programs of Nature (SBS) : the bi-phasic state of the sympaticotonia/parasympaticotonia following the biological conflict (DHS) experienced by the individual at a given moment and it is marked by a series of specific events:

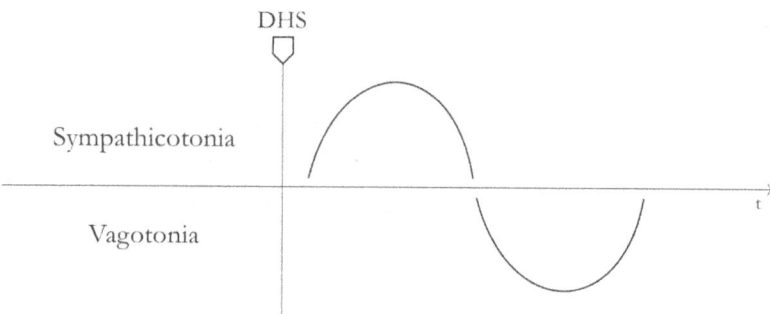

Since DHS has occurred, following a fully meaningful logic from a biological point of view, one can see an activation of the orthosympathetic nervous system: this activation is absolutely optimal to allow the individual to react to that sudden, unexpected event that has caught him off-guard.

The activation of the ortosympathetic system will last until the initial conflict is resolved (DHS). This status of sympathicotonia can be more or less intense (shock mass) depending on the type of conflict experienced. Throughout the sympaticotonia status there will be physic and psychic signs that will show one is in a Conflict-Active phase (CA):

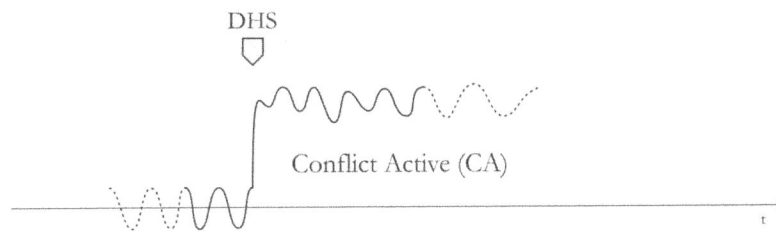

On a psyche level, the person will continue to think about what has happened (obsessive thought), day and night (if it has been particularly intense): this is due to the activation of the sympathethic nervous system.

On a vegetative level, the person will have cold hands and feet, cold skin, lack of appetite, weight loss, insomnia with awakenings between 1 and 3 am and hyperactivity; all this is due to the constant stimulation of the sympathethic nervous system.

On a cerebral level, there will be the formation of the so called Hamer Foci (HH) in specific areas related to the experienced conflict and the corresponding organ. These can be seen during a CAT/CT scan (computerized axial tomography) without contrast.

On an organic level, there will be a structural and functional modification, depending on the embryological origin of the tissue being stimulated by the sympathetic system (3rd Biological Law). During the Active Conflict phase, there are no symptoms (with notably rare exceptions).

This sympathicotonia status following the DHS allows the individual to be able to resolve the conflict in good time (days, weeks or months) and if it happens, this is called Conflictolysis (CL):

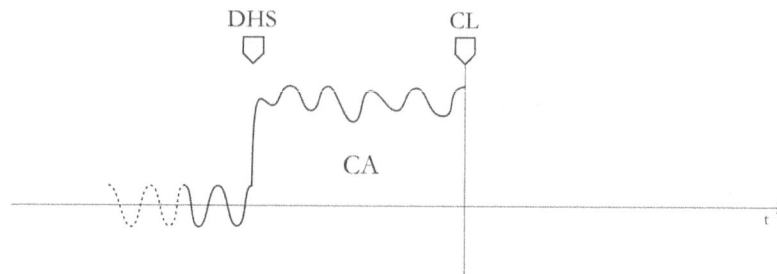

Conflictolysis marks the transition to a second phase, opposite to the first, where there is an activation of the parasympathethic nervous system or vagotonia.

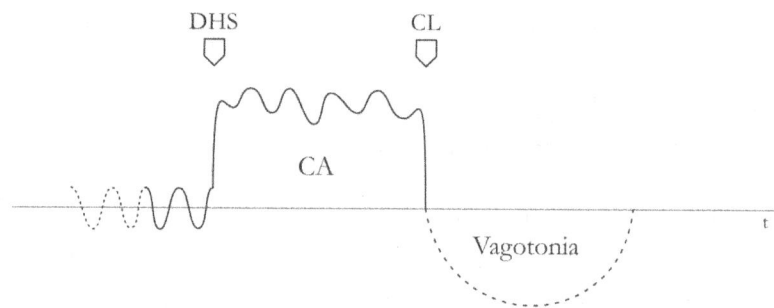

This second vagotonic phase is composed of a phase called A (PCL-A Post-Conflictolysis A), a sympathicotonic phase or peak (Epileptoid Crisis, CE) and a phase B (PCL-B or Post-Conflictolysis B). The duration of this phase is related to the duration of the Conflict-Active phase:

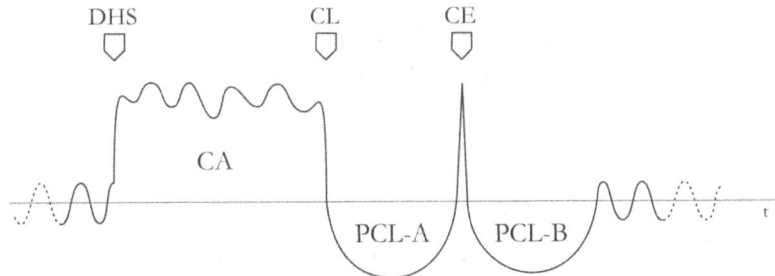

Throughout the vagotonic status, I will have physic and psychic symptoms that will indicate that I am in a PCL (Post-Conflictolysis) status, also called Healing Phase.

On a psyche level, one will no longer think of the event occurred, as this is now settled and remote, and one will be very calm.

On a vegetative level, one will have: warm hands and feet, fatigue.

On a cerebral level, the so-called Hamer-Focus (HF) will show a different conformation of the specific areas related to the experienced conflict and the corresponding organ. These can be seen during a CAT scan (computerized axial tomography) without contrast.

On an organic level, there will be a structural and functional modification,it being the opposite of the sympathicotonic phase one (3rd Biological Law). At this stage, signs and physical symptoms appear, which are precisely related to the DHS suffered previously.

3rd Biological Law of Nature

The ontogenetically conditioned system of the Significant Biological Special Programs of Nature (SBS)

Each tissue originally stems from one of the three embryonic germ layers called: Endoderm, Mesoderm (old and new), Ectoderm (see Appendix); every single tissue derived from a specific embryonic germ layer is subject to a stimulation of the autonomic nervous system (sympathicotonia-parasympathicotonia) and can be subject to one of the four different structural and functional alterations:

- Tissue increase (proliferation)

- Tissue reduction (necrosis, ulceration)

- Increased tissue function (hyperfunction)

- Reduced tissue function (hypofunction)

All the tissues that are derived from Endoderm, in the sympathicotonic phase (CA) will have a tissue and function increase, while in the parasympaticotonic phase (PCL) they will have a loss of function and tissue:

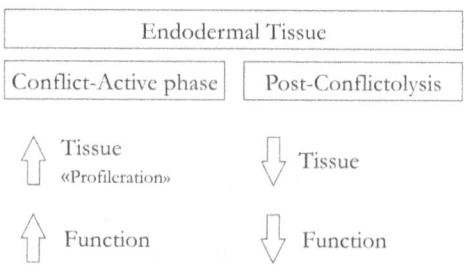

All the tissues that derive from Old Mesoderm, in the sympathicotonic phase (CA) will have a tissue and function increase, while in the parasympathicotonic phase (PCL) they will have a loss of function and tissue:

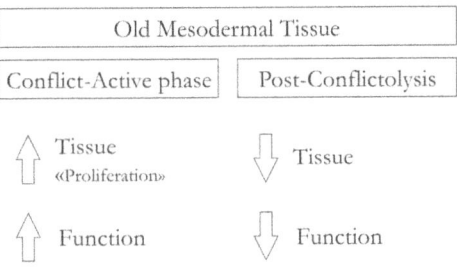

All the tissues deriving from New Mesoderm, in the sympathicotonic phase (CA) will have a loss of tissue and function, while in the parasympathicotonic phase (PCL) they will have an increase of function and tissue:

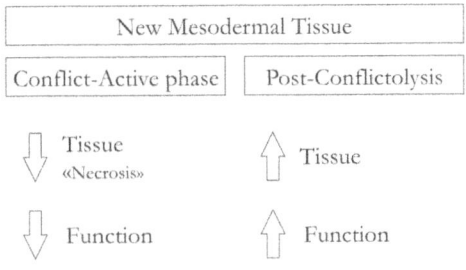

All the tissues that come from Ectoderm, in the sympathicotonic phase (CA) face a loss of tissue and function, while in the parasympathicotonic phase (PCL) they face an increase of function and tissue:

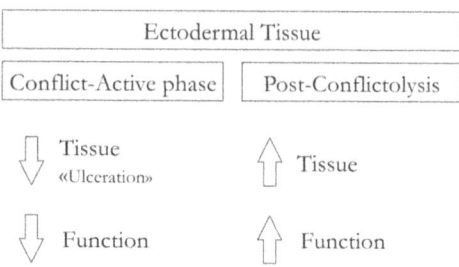

4th Biological Law of Nature

The genetically determined microbial system in the History of Evolution.

Fungi, bacteria and viruses are actively involved in the 2nd phase of the bi-phasic curve (PCL), optimizing the resolution phase.

Endodermal Tissue	Mesodermal Tissue	Ectodermal Tissue

Fungi, Mycobacteria	

	Bacteria	

		Virus

The **Fungi and Mycobacteria** (TBC) participate in the reduction of the tissue deriving from Endoderm that in the active phase (CA) was increased or they do a caseification only during the post-conflict phase. The mycobacteria can also be found in some tissues derived from Old Mesoderm.

The **Bacteria** that derive from Mesoderm proliferate in the active phase (CA) and optimize the tissue healing phase (PCL)

The **Viruses** are in the tissues that derive from Ectoderm in PCL phase and optimize the reconstruction process, restoring the structure.

5th Biological Law of Nature

The quintessence

The 5th biological law reminds us that the Significant Biological Special Programs of Nature (SBS) activated with a DHS have a specific biological sense to ensure the survival of the individual or of the group.

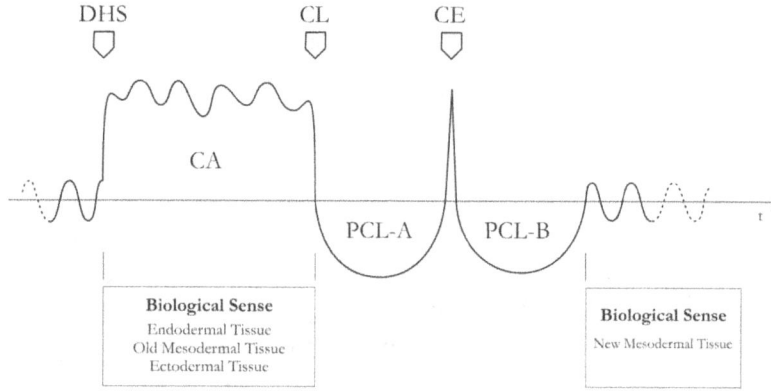

The biological sense is for all tissues in the Active Conflict phase, except for tissues that derive from the New Mesoderm, directed by the White Matter, in which it occurs at the end of the healing phase (normotoni).

3. BIOLOGICAL CONFLICTS

Among all the events that a person experiences, only some will represent a DHS. These are all those conflicts in which the following conditions occur:

- o unexpected

- o sudden

- o acute

- o dramatic

- o experienced in isolation

They are called Biological Conflicts as the occurring event represents a "biological difficulty" which the individual has to overcome and respond to, in order to ensure its biological integrity, survival or integrity of the group to which it belongs:

The reaction is automatic, immediate, instinctive and not mediated by ego; only these conflicts can be called biological and are the only ones that will allow to start the Significant Special Biological Program (SBS); completely different from those conflicts, in Psychology, in which conflict is a clash between what a person desires and his/her inner/interpersonal needs and this clash doesn't allow the satisfaction of this desire, of the need itself or of the objective related to that desire: these are certainly inconveniences for the individual, but will not be capable of causing the activation of a Significant Biological Special Program.

The biological conflicts that can issue a DHS, are the following:

- o "Morsel" conflicts
- o "Attack" conflicts (or fear of being attacked)
- o "Self-Devaluation" conflicts
- o "Territory and Separation" conflicts

Only these conflicts and only if experienced as DHS by the individual (unexpected, sudden, dramatic and lived in isolation) will cause functional and tissue alterations as a significant answer, following the trend of the biphasic curve and the 3rd Biological Law.

Conflicts and the Significant Biological Special Program (SBS) that are produced, allow us both as individuals and as a species to survive in worst-case scenarios and in less dramatic cases to react to the unexpected occurred event.

"Morsel" conflict

These conflicts are related to the survival of the individual, of his species and the maintenance of vital functions: eating, digesting, assimilating, eliminating, evacuating, breathing, hearing and reproduction.

The morsel conflict, with all its variants, involves all the tissues that derive from Endoderm, that is to say from that embryonic germ layer directly involved in preserving the body's vital functions; these are the tissues:

- o Oral Submucosa
- o Palate
- o Parotid Glands
- o Sublingual Salivary Glands

o Tonsils
o Naso-Pharynx
o Lacrimal glands
o Iris
o Thyroid Gland
o Neurohypophysis
o Middle ear
o Eustachian tube
o Esophagus *(lower third only)*
o Lung alveoli
o Stomach *(greater curvature only)*
o Duodenum *(except for duodenal bulb)*
o Liver parenchyma *(no bile ducts nor cholecyst)*
o Pancreas parenchyma *(except for pancreatic ducts and Langerhans islets)*
o Small and large intestine *(Colon)*
o Tongue
o Sigmoid and Rectum *(upper third)*
o Bladder
o Kidney Collecting Tubules
o Prostate
o Uterus and Fallopian Tubes
o Bartholin's glands
o Smegma glands
o Inner navel
o Nuclei of the Acoustic Nerves

The morsel, which is essential for the survival of the individual, is associated to food as well as air morsel (lung alveoli), light morsel (eye, enteroidea), sound morsel (middle ear), water morsel (kidney collecting tubules).

The emotional contents of the morsel conflicts related to man are, to name just a few:

o conflict of "not being able to digest a morsel"

o conflict of "not being able to swallow a morsel"

o death-fright conflict

o conflict of "inability to catch a morsel"

For a detailed study of conflicts relating to DHS , may the reader view the Scientific Table of Germanic New Medicine® (Ed.Amici di Dirk).

"Attack" Conflicts (or fear of being attacked)

These conflicts are related to feeling attacked by everything surrounding the individual, feeling one's own integrity attacked.

The conflict of feeling attacked, with all its variants, involves all tissues that derive from Old Mesoderm, the embryonic germ layer directly concerned with the protection of the individual; these are the tissues:

- ○ Corium Skin *(Dermis)*
- ○ Breast Glands (milk producing glands), *except for ducts*
- ○ Pericardium *(sac containing the heart)*
- ○ Pleura *(lining of the lungs)*
- ○ Peritoneum *(membrane lining of the abdominal cavity and abdominal organs)*
- ○ Greater Omentum

The emotional contents of Attack conflicts (or fear of being attacked) related to man are, to name just a few:

- ○ Conflict of rejecting contact
- ○ Conflict of attack to one's integrity
- ○ Conflict of personal disfigurement
- ○ Conflict of attack against one's heart

For a detailed study of conflicts relating to DHS, the reader is kindly invited to view the Scientific Table of Germanic New Medicine® .

Conflict of "Self-Devaluation"

These conflicts are related to feeling devaluated, fear of failing, not feeling adequate, not being good at doing something, not being up to scratch.

The self-devaluation conflict, with all its variables, involves all the tissues that derive from New Mesoderm, that is to say that embryonic germ layer involved in the individual's growth and strengthening of the group; these are the derived tissues:

- o **Bones** *(including tooth dentin)*
- o Cartilage
- o Tendons and Ligaments
- o Connective tissue
- o Fat tissue
- o Lymphatic system *(Lymph vessels & Lymphnodes)*
- o Blood vessels *(except coronary vessels)*
- o **Muscles** *(striated musculature)*
- o Myocardium *(80% striated heartmuscle)*
- o Kidney Parenchyma
- o Adrenal cortex
- o Spleen
- o Ovaries
- o Testicles

The emotional contents of the devaluation conflicts related to the individual are, to name just a few:

- o Conflict of intellectual devaluation
- o Conflict of not being adequate
- o Conflict of incapability to escape a situation
- o Conflict of feeling left outside a situation
- o Conflict of having lost someone
- o Conflict of being tied to a ball and chain

For a detailed study of conflicts relating to DHS , may the reader view the Scientific Table of Germanic New Medicine®.

"Territorial and Separation" conflicts

These conflicts are related to the group to which one belongs, to the territory and separation. The territorial conflict (fight and separation), with all its variants, involves all tissues that stem from Ectoderm, that is to say that embryonic germ layer directly connected to territorial fight and separation. These are the tissues stemming from the ectoderm:

- o Epidermis *(skin)*
- o Periosteum *(skin that covers the bones)*
- o Mouth *(upper mucosa)*, incl. palate, gums, tongue, lining of salivary gland ducts
- o Nasal and sinuses membrane
- o Inner ear
- o Lens, cornea, conjunctiva, retina, and vitreous body of the eyes
- o Teeth enamel
- o Lining of the milk ducts
- o Lining of the thyroid gland ducts and of pharyngeal ducts
- o Lining of the heart vessels *(coronary arteries and coronary veins)*
- o Esophagus *(upper 2/3)*
- o Laryngeal mucosa and Bronchial mucosa
- o Stomach lining *(small curvature)*
- o Lining of the bile ducts and gall bladder, and of pancreatic ducts
- o Cervix and vagina
- o Lining of renal pelvis, bladder, ureter, and urethra
- o Lining of the rectum *(lower part)*
- o Nerve cells of the Central Nervous System

The emotional contents of territorial conflicts related to man are, to name just a few :

- o Territorial conflict
- o Territorial threatening conflict
- o Territorial anger conflict
- o Conflict of inability of marking the territory
- o Separation conflict

o   Conflict of having no right to bite

For a detailed study of conflicts relating to DHS may the reader refer to the Scientific Table of Germanic New Medicine®.

Andrea Taddei

4. THE "CONFLICT-ACTIVE" PHASE

The DHS that occurred marks the beginning of the Significant Biologic Special program of Nature. The sympathethic nervous system will be activated to bring a response to the event, which occurred so suddenly and unexpectedly, in order to solve it as soon as possible: this phase is called Conflict-Active (CA).

The individual in a Conflict-Active phase will continue to mull all day long over that event that occurred so unexpectedly and, if this event has been very intense, the person will think about it also during the night and wake up between 1 and 3 am. On a somatic level,the individual will have very cold hands and feet, lack of appetite, hyperactivity, mild fatigue.

During the Conflict-Active phase, the individual is fine and has no symptoms that can worry him, all his physical and mental energies are directed to solve his problem (DHS). Other smaller problems are momentarily put aside and, in any case, they are not a priority at this time.

In this phase, depending on the type of conflict (DHS) experienced by the individual, the tissues begin to "respond" to the sympathicotonia status but there are no symptoms:

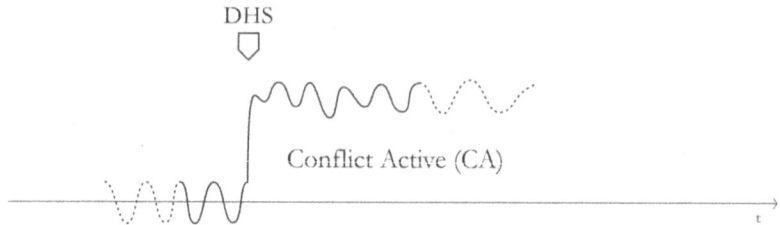

If DHS is related to a morsel conflict corresponding to a tissue that derives from Endoderm, in the Conflict-Active phase, the tissue will increase (proliferation) and its related function will increase as well:

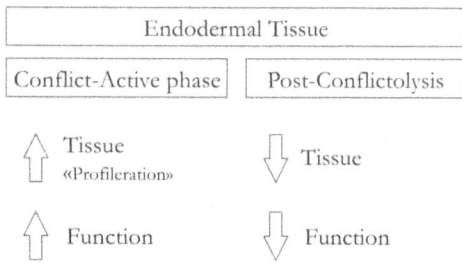

If DHS is related to an attack conflict corresponding to a tissue that derives from Old Mesoderm, in the Conflict-Active phase, the tissue will increase and its related function will increase as well:

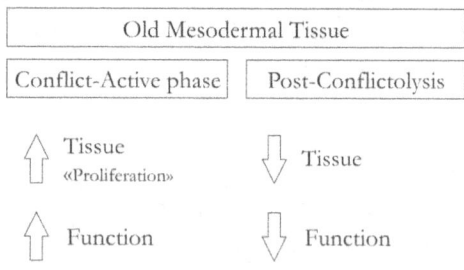

If DHS is related to a self-devaluation conflict corresponding to a tissue that derives from New Mesoderm, in the Conflict-Active phase, the tissue will be reduced and so will its related function:

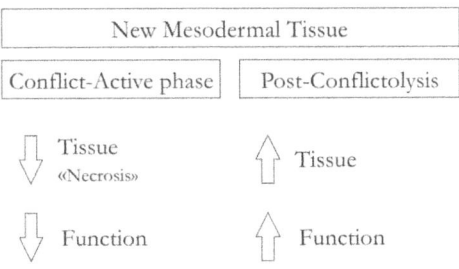

If DHS is related to a territorial conflict corresponding to a tissue that comes from Endoderm, in the Conflict Active phase, the tissue will be reduced (ulceration) and so will its function:

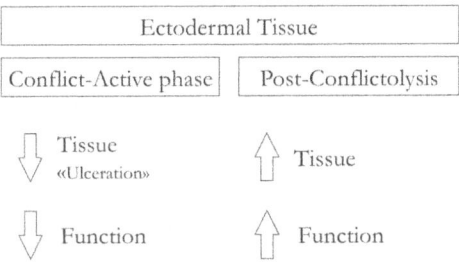

The biological sense (5th Biological Law) for all conflicts that derive from Endoderm, from Old Mesoderm and Ectoderm is in the Conflict-Active phase:

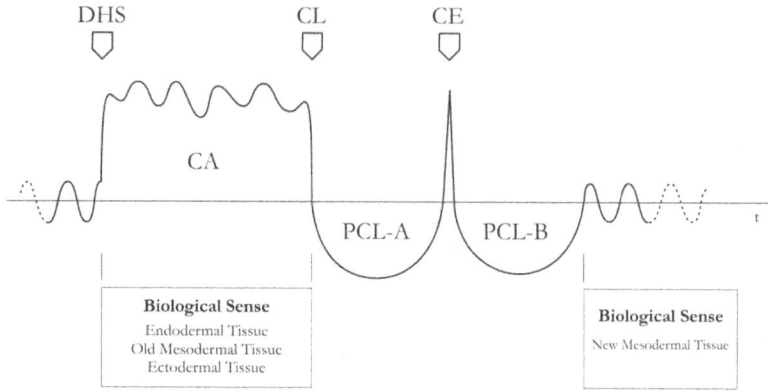

5. CONFLICTOLYSIS

Conflictolysis occurs when, thanks to the state of sympathicotonia, I have been in, I am able to resolve the conflict (DHS). The resolution of the conflict can happen in different ways, more or less depending on the individual; one can manage to finally get away from what has happened, one can deal with the situation or, it may occur, circumstances spontaneously evolve in a better direction even without one's direct intervention:

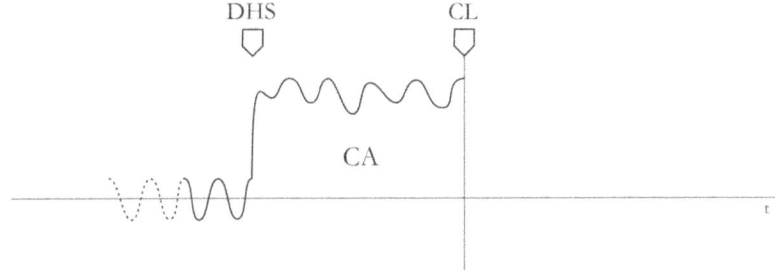

Conflictolysis is an event that allows the resolution of a biological conflict, has a positive connotation, it represents a relief, a solution.

After Conflictolysis, a phase change occurs; from a status of ortosympathicotonia, a parasympathicotonia or vagotonic phase will appear and this is called Post-Conflictolysis phase of resolution.

Andrea Taddei

6. POST-CONFLICTOLYSIS PHASE

The Healing phase - Post Conflictolysis (PCL) represents the second phase of the biphasic curve; the autonomic nervous system switches from activation of the sympathetic to an activation of the parasympathetic:

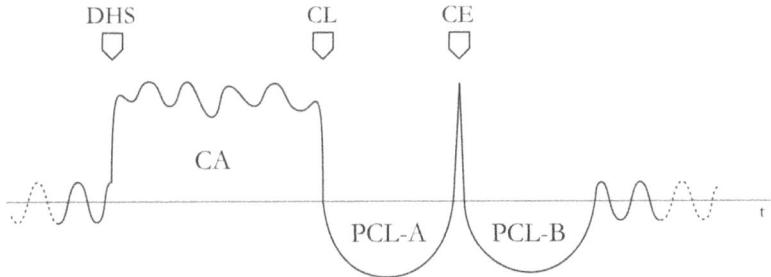

In this vagotonic phase, the individual will be tired and will sleep longer than usual if possible, he will no longer think of his problem because it is finally solved and at a somatic level he will have warm hands, feet and skin and he will see signs and symptoms that will prompt him to a medical consultation to give a name to his "disease". The symptoms that occur in this phase are related to the type of DHS occurred earlier and which started the Significant Biological Special program: a cold, bronchitis, vitiligo, dermatitis, gastritis, hepatitis, cystitis, psoriasis, pleurisy, conjunctivitis, myopia, low back pain, rhinitis, headache, arthritis… and all the so-called "diseases" that have a precise and unique correspondence with a biological

conflict (DHS)
In this second phase called vagotonic, the tissues begin to respond to the parasympathicotonic phase (3rd Biological Law):

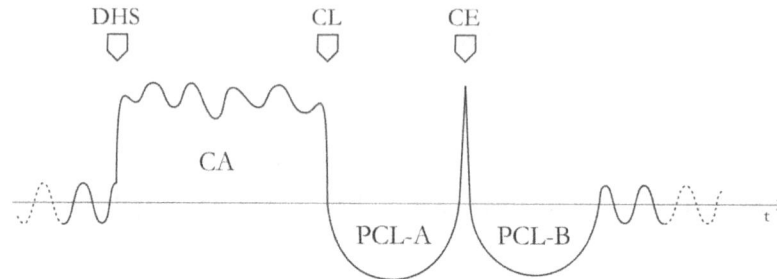

If DHS is related to a morsel conflict, that corresponds to any tissue that derives from Endoderm in resolution, the tissue and its function will be reduced:

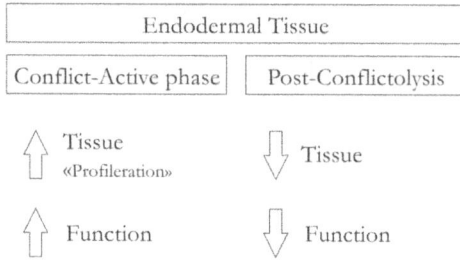

If DHS is related to a attack conflict, that corresponds to any tissue that derives from Old Mesoderm in resolution, the tissue and its function will be reduced:

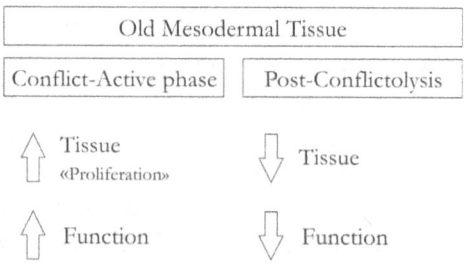

If DHS is related to a devaluation conflict, corresponding to any tissue deriving from the New Mesoderm in resolution, the tissue and its function will end this phase with a surplus of tissue:

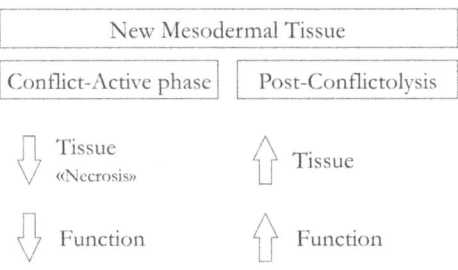

If DHS is related to a territorial conflict, that corresponds to any tissue that derives from Ectoderm in resolution, the tissue and its function will be replenished:

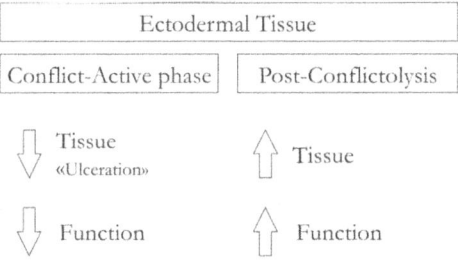

As you can see in this picture, the vagotonic resolution phase is composed by three curves:

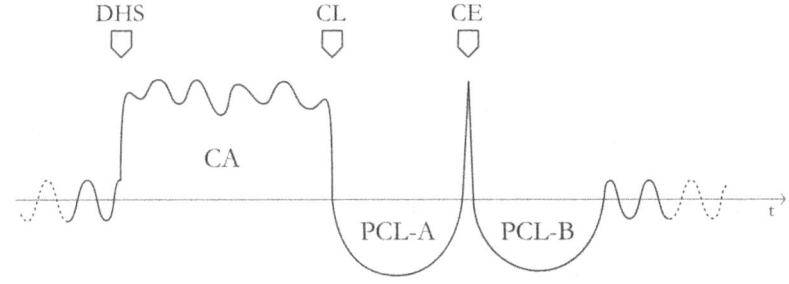

The PCL A (Post-Conflictolysis phase A) is the first parasympathicotonic in which one or more symptoms appear. Analysing a single biphasic curve and without conflict relapses, the temporal duration of this phase is exactly half the duration of the Conflict-Active phase but with a maximum duration of 3 weeks (e.g.):

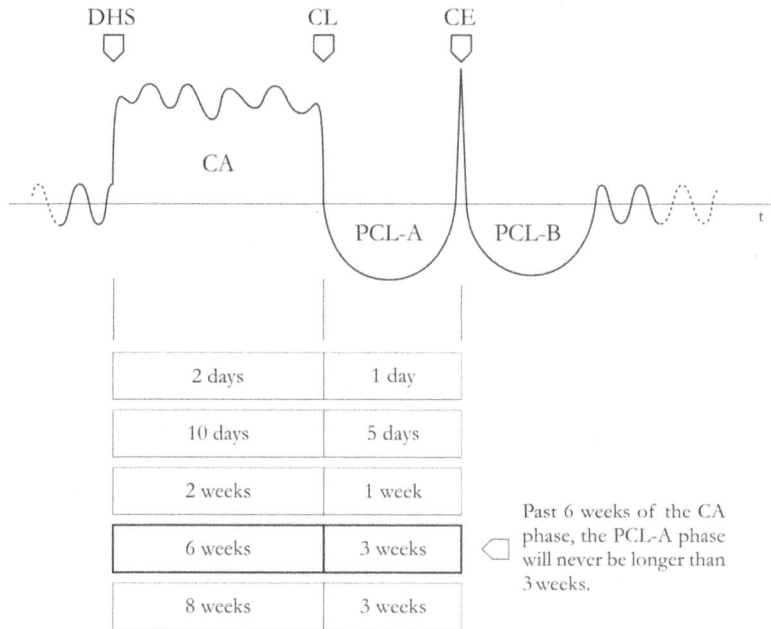

2 days	1 day
10 days	5 days
2 weeks	1 week
6 weeks	3 weeks
8 weeks	3 weeks

Past 6 weeks of the CA phase, the PCL-A phase will never be longer than 3 weeks.

If the CA phase lasted two weeks, the PCL A phase has a duration of one week. Past 6 weeks of the CA phase, the PCL A phase will never be longer than 3 weeks).

After the PCL A phase, a sympathicotonic peak is shown, which is called EPILEPTOID CRISIS (EPI-CRISIS) (EC) (If DHS is motorial, it will be called Epileptic crisis). This sympathicotonic peak occurs in the middle of the healing phase and its function is to reduce the brain edema at the HH level : it will be associated to very intense and acute symptoms called renal colic, biliary colic, intestinal colic, panic attack (and more) but it will always be in relation to the emotional content of the initial DHS.

Biologically, the epi-crysis has a duration that can range from 10 -20 seconds to 4 hours:

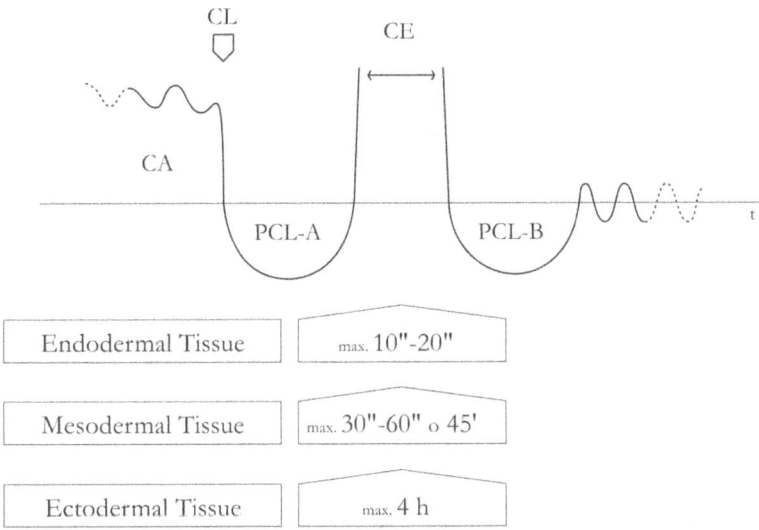

The duration of the Epi-crysis, it often happens, can exceed maximum if it enters a "hanging" phase.

At the end of the Epileptoid crisis a vagotonic phase will recur, called PCL B, with less intense symptoms, which will mark the end of the Significant Biological special Program of Nature before getting back to normotonia:

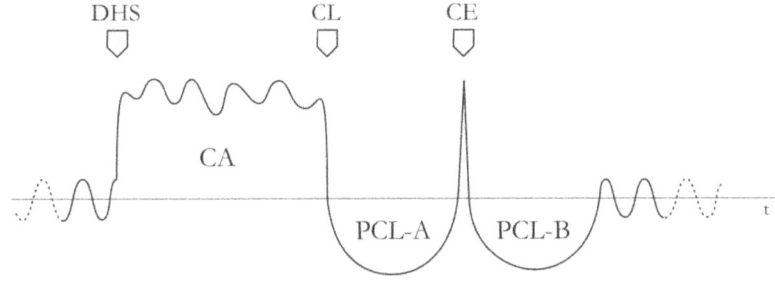

During the Post-Conflictolysis phase, besides having the specific symptoms determined by the DHS and the type of tissue involved, one may also run a temperature of varying degrees, depending on the embryonic derivation of tissue:

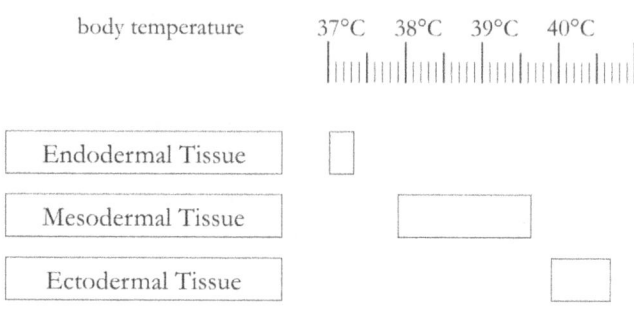

The biological sense (5th Biological Law) for tissues that derive from the new Mesoderm comes at the end of the bi-phasic curve, when normotonia is restored:

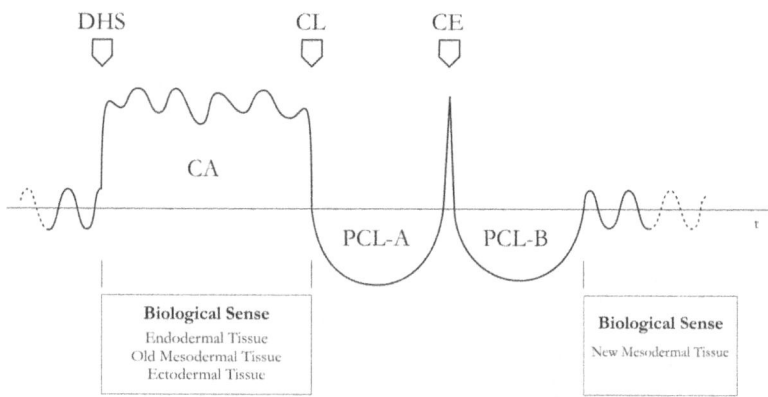

7. A BIOLOGICAL VISION

*"Things get logical
when one understands them"*

Now we can better understand what occurred to me in the beginning: At a certain stage of my life I live a dramatic situation, suddenly, it catches me off-guard, I never thought such a thing could happen to me, in that very moment, I am speechless, I am bewildered (DHS).

I'm freezing, my hands are very cold, and for the following minutes, days, hours I can't help thinking of what happened to me, so intensely, so unexpectedly, I cannot think of anything else, I say to myself, I want to sort this thing out! But now I can't, I keep thinking about how to get out, I do not sleep these nights, I always wake up around 2 or 3 am.(**Conflict-Active phase**, CA)

I found the solution! I will do such and such, settle everything now! I'm going to fix it (**Conflictolysis**, CL)

I've just got back, I am happy, I feel relieved at last! But now I'm a little tired, I am nearly going to bed without eating, what a hard time I have been through! Today has been a busy day!

The day after

I did not hear the alarm, it is eleven o'clock am, but I'm really tired, I feel I'm running a temperature, my body aches, especially my legs, I cannot even get up, as if a truck had run me over.

This makes me want to laugh as it's always like this…we experience an acute, dramatic, unexpected situation and when it is resolved, symptoms come out, but what makes me really laugh even more is that it's always been that way, I just did not understand and no one ever described this relationship between cause and effect to me, until now.

What we have always called "disease" is just the sane and significant response to a particular event that occurred time ago.

We were taught that when we have a symptom, there is necessarily something wrong.

Biologically instead, when a symptom appears, and with it, the pain or the symptom, it is right to know that one finds oneself in a resolution phase. Our tissue is in resolution and it is taking, provided that all goes well, the right time to repair, with confidence, what has changed for basic needs in the Conflict-Active phase.

8. LATERALITY

It is fundamental to know whether you are right- or left-handed to understand how the individual functions.

Of all the tests that can be done to determine whether you are right-handed or left-handed, Dr. Hamer was able to verify that the only suitable one to establish the exact laterality is the one of applause.

By applauding like in a theater, the hand that beats above gives dominance: the right-handed individual will hit his right hand over the left while the left-handed will hit his left hand over the right one.

In right-handed people, both male and female, the non-dominant side, the left one ,is related to the nest, to their mother and their children or animals. The right side applies to all other figures (father, husband, lover, friend, friends, girl-friends, employer, in-laws ...):

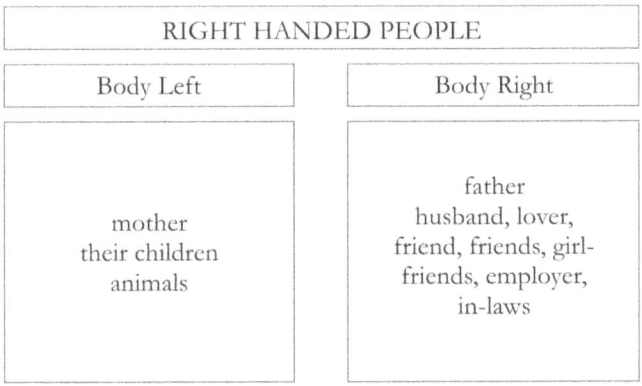

RIGHT HANDED PEOPLE	
Body Left	Body Right
mother their children animals	father husband, lover, friend, friends, girl-friends, employer, in-laws

In left-handed people, both male and female, the non-dominant side, the right one, is in relation to their mother and their children, or animals, while the dominant regards all other persons:

LEFT HANDED PEOPLE	
Body Left	Body Right
father husband, lover, friend, friends, girl- friends, employer, in-laws	mother their children animals

The rule of laterality applies only to tissues that derive from Mesoderm and Ectoderm.

9. HANGING HEALINGS

When a DHS occurs, the individual goes from a Conflict-Active phase (CA) to a Conflictolysis and then a vagotonic Post-Conflictolysis phase starts and will return, with its biologic time, to a normotonia.

We call it "hanging healing" when the individual, instead of progressing to the biphasic curve, as described, will keep going from one vagotonic phase (PCL) to a sympathicotonic one (CA), not necessarily returning to normotonia.

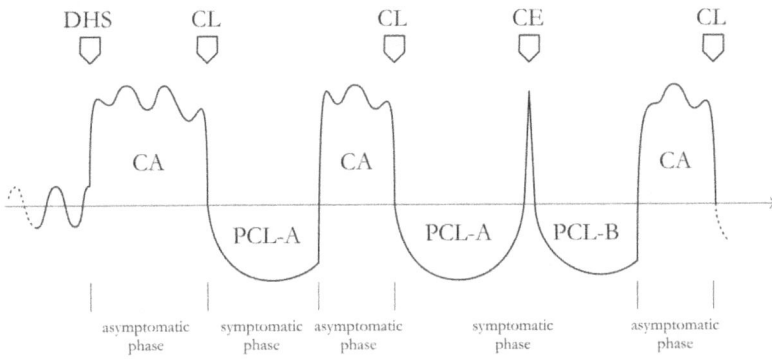

This pattern is due to the fact that, when one is in a vagotonic phase of CA, the event occurs again bringing one back into a conflict-active phase. This trend can last long, even for months. As to symptoms, they will show in a vagotonic phase (PCL) and then one will experience a fading or disappearance of symptoms in the sympathycotonic phase (CA).

49

Andrea Taddei

10. CONFLICT RELAPSES OR "TRACKS"

At the exact time DHS occurs, our nervous system records not only the conflict that will trigger the Significant Biologic Special Program but also all those "signals" that accompanied the DHS.

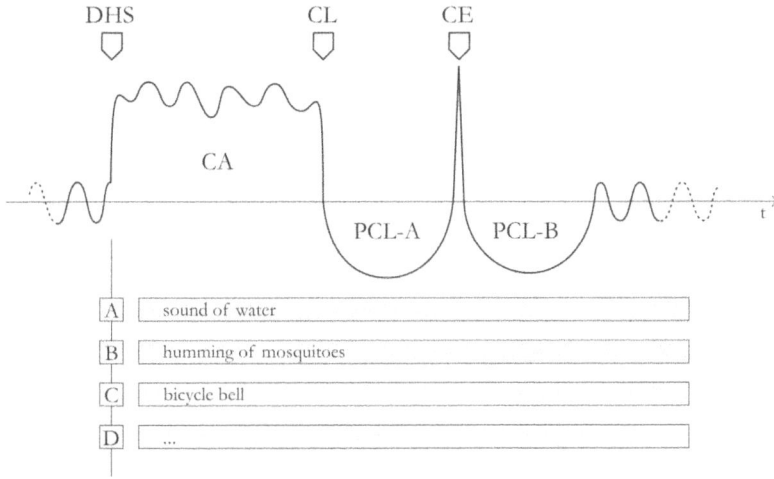

If a DHS of any kind occurs while I am walking on a riverside, in addition to the DHS I will fix a series of "signs", for example, the sound of water, the humming of mosquitoes , the local temperature, the bicycle bell and so on. These "signals" in future, if reappearing all together or isolated from one another, will reactivate the original biphasic curve related to the event previously experienced years before; if this occurs, as an effect, I will see symptoms showing in relation to the curve.

This mode, from a biological point of view, is optimal because it is a "warning signal" to prevent one from bumping into such a peculiar situation that has already occurred.

11. REFUGEE CONFLICT

Whenever one experiences DHS, a new Biological Program (SBS) begins, so if one has different DHS at the same time, one will have different bi-phasic curves, some in an active phase and some in resolution:

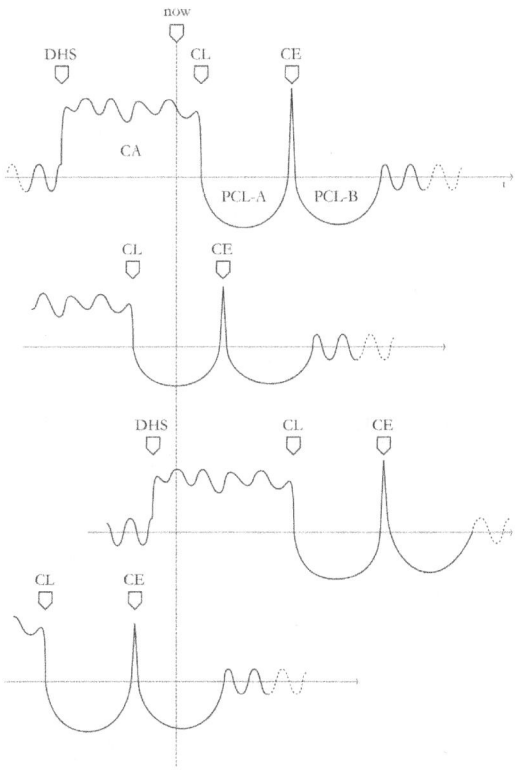

This means that, in a given moment, one will be in CA for one or more DHS, in PCL-A for one or more DHS and in PCL-B for one or more other DHS.

So: for the conflicts I will be having in CA, I will show no symptoms but I will not sleep at night and will feel anxiety.

Instead, I will have a particularly annoying symptom about the conflict in the PCL A phase and a different symptom for the PCL B phase of the DHS that I am living, but at least for this latter conflict in the solution phase I am much calmer and the worst is over.

Among all the biological conflicts we are having, there is a very important and essential one, for its practical implications that can increase, if it is active, the symptomatic manifestation of the parasympatheticotonic curve (PCL-A and B) as well as of any bi-phasic curve related to an active SBS.

This is the refugee conflict, a program of water retention, related to the system of kidney collecting tubules (derivating from Endoderm) that in the Conflict-Active phase, increase their function:

Endodermal Tissue	
Conflict-Active phase	Post-Conflictolysis

⇧ Tissue «Profileration»   ⇩ Tissue

⇧ Function   ⇩ Function

During the sympathicotonic phase of the kidney collecting tubules:

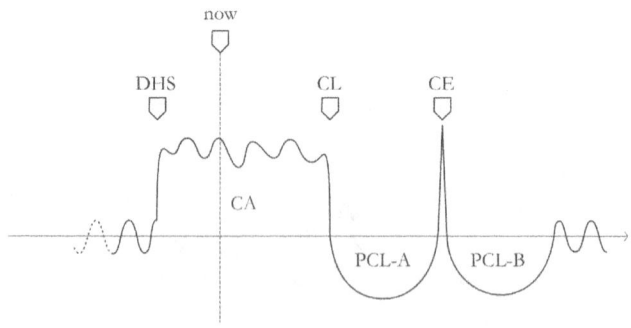

I will experience systemic water retention (the whole body will feel bloated): I will feel bloated, not necessarily with other symptoms, but if in addition to the SBS of collecting tubules(active refugee conflict) I also have another SBS in a solution A phase (PCL-A), the symptoms of this conflict will increase exponentially.

The result will be a local edema of the 2nd curve plus global edema (CA of the kidney collecting tubules) of the 1st curve and this will cause more serious symptoms (local edema + global edema = more pain or symptom):

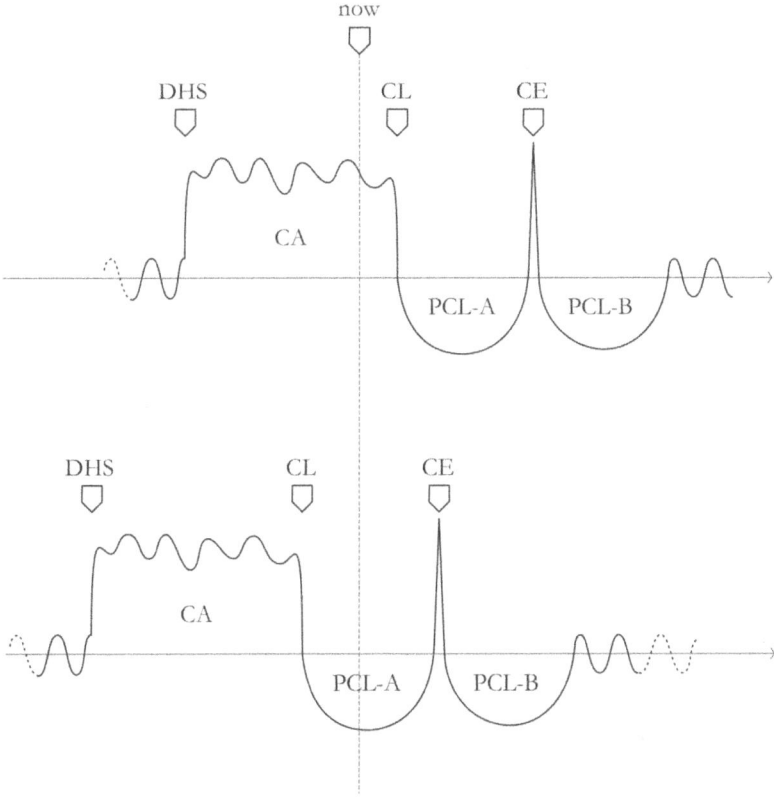

A single healing curve (PCL) gives an ache or a symptom that can reach 2-3 in a range from 1 to 10. Together with an active refugee conflict, the ache goes up to 7-8.

Andrea Taddei

12. HEADACHE

Involved organ: **bone or muscle of the cranial vault**
Embryologic derivation: **New Mesoderm**
Active cerebral areas: **relay of the Cerebral Medulla**
Conflict: **intellectually devaluated**

The related **Biological Conflict** is the following: I feel intellectually devaluated; I am not able, I can't do something, someone told me I did something wrong, but this is always on an intellectual level. The are quite many situations where an intellectual devalutation conflict can occur: at school, at work, in the family, with friends.

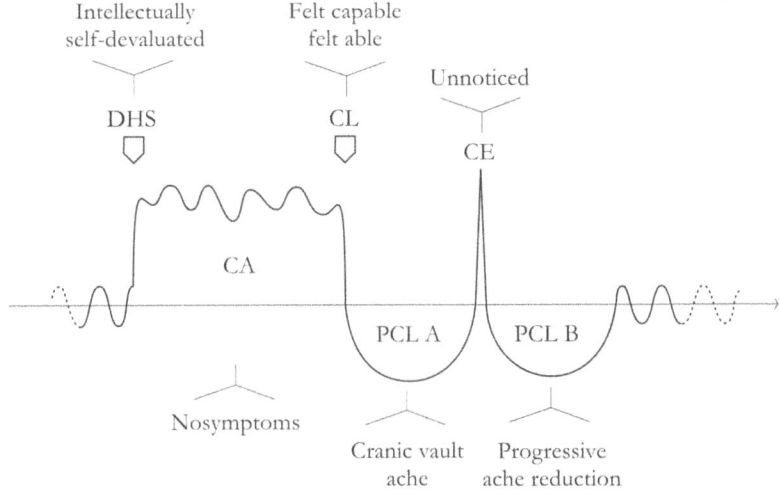

Conflict-Active phase (CA): I have no symptoms, but I feel worried and pensive, I dwell (sympathicotonia) on the conflict.

Conflictolysis CL: I felt capable, I felt able, I could do it or, the person who disparaged me before, now recognizes the mistake and has reconsidered me.

Post-Conflictolysis A (PCLA): the cranic vault ache is strong but bearable (maximum 3 out of 10), on the right or left side according to the laterality rule. If in the meantime I am dealing with a Refugee Active conflict, I'll have an unbearable ache (9-10 out of 10). Great fatigue, prostration (parasympaticotonia)

Epi-Crysis (CE): for some tissues that derive from the new Mesoderm, the epi-crysis goes on unnoticed.

In **Post-Conflictolysis B** (PCLB): progressive ache reduction, which already started at the end of the PCLA,

Normotonia: absence of ache

In-depth addendum

If the duration between DHS and CL was 4 days, the symptom healing phase (PCLA) will last two days.

If I am right-handed and I lived a conflict at school for a passed exam, my headache will be on the right side of the cranic vault (see chapter 7 – laterality)

If there are some hanging healings, one will frequently have headaches and intermittent relief (CA solution- see chapter 8-hanging healings).

APPENDIX

The Nervous System

The nervous system is anatomically organized as follows:

- **Central Nervous System** (CNS) which comprises the encephalon (brain) and spinal cord (neuraxis): it receives, integrates, and processes the afferent stimuli coming from the Peripheral Nervous System(PNS) which in turn receives the efferent stimuli from the CNS.
- **Peripheral Nervous System** (PNS) consists of cranial nerves and spinal nerves stemming from the spinal cord and it is divided in two main parts:
  - **Somatic Nervous System** (SNS) controlling voluntary responses.
  - **Autonomic Nervous System** (ANS), in charge of involuntary responses, consisting of:
    - **Parasympathetic Nervous System**
    - **Sympathetic Nervous System**

The Autonomic Nervous System, in addition to regulating the homeostasis of the organism, controls all functions of the body that are not normally under conscious control; innervating every tissue, organ and bowel, this system cannot be influenced by will and functions with autonomous mechanisms but still in close mutual collaboration with the Central Nervous System.

The orthosympathetic innervation is traditionally described as a component that performs an escape/attack alert function, mobilizes and organizes energy resources in an emergency or in danger, stimulates the heart and lungs, dilates the bronchi, contracts the arteries and inhibits the digestive system; it prepares the body for physical activity, while the parasympathetic system is a system that allows saving energy, digestion, sleep and rest.

Embriologial Layers

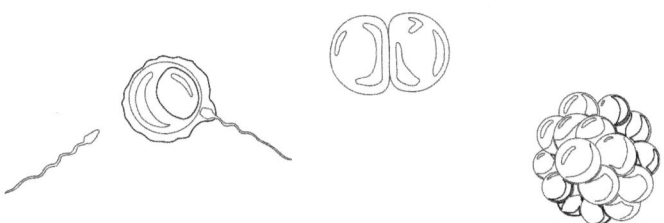

The fertilized cell (zygote) through processes of division, differentiation and growth will generate the fetus.

Embryonic development goes through several stages of segmentation (morula, blastocysts), gastrulation and organogenesis.

In gastrulation, the cells are distributed in three layers of tissue:

- Endoderm
- Mesoderm
- Ectoderm

By subsequent differentiation, all tissues of the body are generated. At the 8th week of gestation, embryonic development is completed to begin organogenesis and the embryo is now called fetus.

About the author

Andrea Taddei (*Milan 1970, Italy*), during the period of his study at the University of Medicine, he learns also different bio-disciplines such as Craniosacral Therapy, Traditional Chinese Medicine, Shiatsu, Ayurvedic Medicine, Yoga and Meditation. Following the abandonment of Academic studies, he devoted full time to the diffusion and study of Craniosacral Therapy. He holds educational seminars and advanced courses on the 5 Biological Laws in Italy and abroad. The reference site is: www.5biologicallaws.com

Andrea Taddei